Ageless Beauty
with
Herbal Secrets

Revitalize Your Skin. Defy aging, Boost Your Confidence with a Radiant Look.

Dr Arundhati Hoskeri

Ageless Beauty
with
Herbal Secrets

Dr Arundhati Hoskeri

Publication: December 2023

All Rights Reserved.

Copyright @ Dr Arundhati Hoskeri

No part of this publication can be reproduced, copied, or transmitted in any form or by any means without the author's permission.

Email: ah1478670@gmail.com

Disclaimer

This book, "Ageless Beauty with Herbal Secrets," is a guide to exploring the world of homemade skincare solutions using natural ingredients. While the information provided is based on traditional practices and herbal remedies, it is important to note that individual skin types may react differently to various ingredients. It is important to note that the author and publisher, who are not licensed skincare professionals, base the information in this book on traditional practices and herbal remedies.

Readers are encouraged to conduct patch tests and consult with dermatologists or healthcare professionals before incorporating new skincare routines or products, especially if they have **pre-existing skin conditions or allergies.** The recipes and techniques presented in this book are not to be taken as a substitute for professional medical advice, diagnosis, or treatment.

The author and publisher do not claim any liability for the outcomes of the skincare practices detailed in this book. It is recommended that readers exercise caution, use their discretion, and modify recipes based on personal preferences and sensitivities.

The effectiveness and results of herbal remedies may vary for individuals. It is advisable to approach skincare as a holistic practice, incorporating a **balanced diet, regular**

exercise, and proper hydration alongside any topical treatments.

By choosing to engage with the content of this book, readers acknowledge and accept the inherent risks associated with experimenting with homemade skincare products. Ultimately, the pursuit of ageless beauty is a personal journey, and this book serves as a gentle guide, empowering individuals to make informed decisions about their skincare routines.

Dr Arundhati Govind Hoskeri

Disclaimer 4

Link to My Books Published in the Series: Natural Medicine and Alternative Healing 9

A Gift for You 10

Book Overview 11

About The Author 14

Chapter 1 18

"From Kitchen to Glam: The Pros of Making Your Beauty Goodies" 18

Important Considerations for Skincare 24

Chapter 2 26

"In Tune with Your Skin: A Guide to Skin Type Awareness." 26

Chapter 3: 36

Why do Moisturizers Matter for Our Skin? .. 36

Chapter 4: Unveiling the Secrets of Natural Moisturizers 46

Herbal Moisturizers for Normal Skin Type .. 47

Herbal Moisturizers for Dry Skin 53

Herbal Moisturizers for Oily Skin 59

Moisturizers For Combination Skin 65

Herbal Moisturizers for Sensitive Skin 71

Chapter 5: 79

Homemade Packs for a Radiant Skin 79

    Homemade Face Packs Can Contribute to a Radiant Complexion. 80

    Some Useful Tips for Using Any Face Pack . 84

Chapter 6: 86

Let's Get into Action! DIY Face Packs. 86

    Homemade Moisturizing Face Pack 106

Chapter 7: 108

A Fascinating Story of Lipstick 108

Chapter 8: Homemade Lip balms 113

Chapter 9: 123

Timeless Beauty- Easy-to-Make Anti-Aging Creams 123

Secrets to Delay Wrinkles 127
Homemade Nourishing Night Cream for Face and Neck 131

Benefits of Facial Massage 135
DIY Anti-aging Cream for Massage 140

Step-by-Step Techniques for Facial Massage
.... 142

Chapter 10: Holistic Approach to Glowing Skin
.... 146

References 156

Link to My Books Published in the Series:
Natural Medicine and Alternative Healing

Book 1: Home Remedies for Women's Ailments

https://rxe.me/1PKX9K

Book 2: Healthy Heart with Home Remedies

http://rxe.me/5QWNBK

Book 3: Healthy Skin with Herbal Remedies

http://rxe.me/BFD7KS

Book 4: Skincare Secrets for Flawless Beauty

http://rxe.me/QGM9BV

5. Holistic Secrets to Lustrous Hair

http://relinks.me/B0CL2MCM7N

✶✶✶✶✶✶

A Gift for You

Dear Reader, please click on the link below for instant access.

https://healthy-mind-in-healthy-body.ck.page/2c28568068

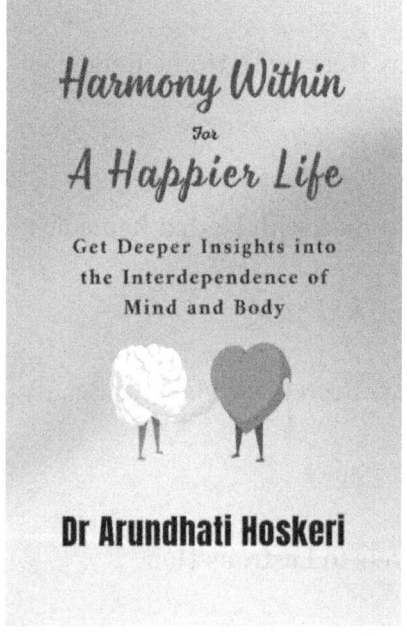

Book Overview

Welcome to the journey of timeless beauty—a guide that uncovers the secrets to making your anti-aging miracles right in the comfort of your home. This book will take you step by step to a radiant and ageless complexion in a world where youthfulness is cherished. Explore the power of nature's bounty as we embark on a venture to create exotic anti-aging creams, rejuvenating face packs, luscious lip balms, and a range of cosmetics designed to defy time.

In these pages, simplicity meets potency as we explore the art of harnessing natural ingredients to nurture and revitalize your skin. No need for complex formulations or mysterious elixirs—just the pure essence of botanical wonders that have stood the test of time.

Whether you're a skincare enthusiast or a novice seeking the elixir of everlasting youth, this book promises a straightforward and empowering journey toward a more radiant, resilient, and age-defying you. Discover the joy of self-care as you delve into the creation of personalized anti-aging solutions that cater to your unique needs. Unleash the transformative potential of ingredients found in your kitchen and embrace the beauty of a holistic approach to skincare. Get ready to redefine aging, one nourishing cream, soothing face pack, and sumptuous lip balm at a time. Your radiant future awaits!

An interesting story behind this book

A couple of decades ago, I participated in a teacher training program in Singapore that drew educators from various corners of the globe. During the initial ice-breaker session on the first day, our trainer spontaneously grouped us into fives, tasking us with gathering as many facts as possible about our group members within a swift three minutes. Subsequently, each of us was tasked with introducing two members from our group to the others.

In my group, there was a young teacher from Korea, Ara, who I thought was in her mid-twenties. Engaging in conversation, she revealed she taught at a high school, spoke English fluently, and astonishingly boasted fifteen years of teaching experience. Struck with awe, I couldn't fathom her age as she possessed a radiant, youthful complexion without a single fine line on her face or neck.

Over the next four days, as we spent time together, my curiosity led me to inquire about Ara's age. To my surprise, she disclosed she was forty-five. Intrigued by her secret to maintaining a youthful appearance, Ara shared she practiced daily meditation, engaged in Pranayama (breathing exercises), and nourished her skin with homemade cosmetics using natural ingredients.

This revelation ignited my curiosity, prompting me to delve into the world of homemade cosmetics.

In the time predating smartphones and the internet's widespread availability, I delved into books, consulted Ayurveda and Naturopathy textbooks, conversed with people, and reflected on the beauty practices passed down from my mother and grandmother.

The culmination of this exploration resulted in creating the books **"Ageless Beauty with Herbal Secrets"** and **"Skincare Secrets for Flawless Beauty"** published in September 2023, which cover everything about face scrubs, body scrubs, toners, moisturizing creams, face packs, lip balms, and face massage, etc.

Ara generously shared some popular recipes from her country that incorporated rice as a key ingredient. Having tried them all, I can attest to their amazing qualities, and I'm confident you'll love them, too.

******

About The Author

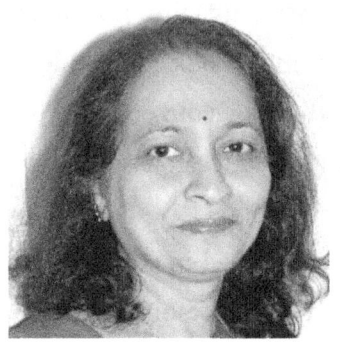

Dr Arundhati G Hoskeri

MSc, MEd, PhD, MA (English), ACTL Diploma in Public Speaking (Trinity College of London)
NDHS (Doctor of Natural Health Sciences)
Certified Cyber Crime Intervention Officer (CCIO)

Educational Consultant for Cambridge International School

Former Director and Principal of Cambridge International School and I B World School

A Lifelong Learner, Author, Poet, passionate Educator, Counsellor, Natural Health Science Expert, Motivational Speaker, and Freelance journalist.

Dr Arundhati Govind Hoskeri is a remarkable individual whose passion for learning and educational commitments has defined her illustrious journey. With an unquenchable thirst for knowledge, she has obtained master's degrees in three distinct subjects, a testament to her dedication to intellectual growth.

Her academic journey culminated in attaining a PhD in education, reflecting her deep-seated desire to contribute meaningfully to the field.

Throughout her impressive career spanning 37 years, Dr. Arundhati has been a trailblazer in education. Her leadership acumen shines through her role as the head of a prestigious IB (International Baccalaureate) World School and Cambridge International School for over two decades.

This extensive experience underscores her exceptional ability to shape the educational landscape and nurture future generations.

Beyond her role as an educator, Dr Arundhati's versatile talents extend into various domains. She is a gifted educator and a practitioner of natural health sciences, earning the title of a Natural Health Science (NDHS) doctor.

Her communication prowess is evident in her ACTL Diploma in Public Speaking from Trinity College of London, which has undoubtedly played a pivotal role in her success as a **speaker, educator, and author.**

Dr Arundhati's impact reaches far beyond the classroom. Her accomplishments as a poet have garnered recognition on national and international platforms, including in countries like India, Sri Lanka, and Malaysia.

Her thought-provoking contributions to journalism have graced the pages of esteemed national and international magazines and newspapers, establishing her as a credible voice on various subjects.

As an avid reader and extensive researcher, Dr Arundhati's intellectual curiosity has resulted in the publication of many research articles in esteemed educational journals and conferences—her ability to combine academia with practical insights positions her as a thought leader in her field.

Her compassion and **dedication to holistic well-being** are evident in her motivational speaker and healer role, where she uses her expertise to promote **alternative medicine and positive transformation**. Accolades and recognition, a testament to her unwavering commitment and exemplary contributions, mark Dr Arundhati's journey.

Her presence as a moderator, keynote speaker, and presenter in national and international seminars has solidified her status as a respected voice in various forums.

Dr Arundhati lends her expertise as a consultant to upcoming and established Cambridge International School, further impacting the educational landscape with her wealth of knowledge.

Notably, her journey as an author takes center stage. With a focus on physical health, mental well-being, and the intricate nuances of human behavior, her writing endeavors are a testament to her dedication to empowering individuals with practical insights and actionable advice.

Dr Arundhati's legacy has a profound impact and unwavering dedication. Her multifaceted contributions to education, physical and mental health, writing, and motivational speaking continue to inspire and uplift individuals across the globe, shining brightly through her accomplishments and sincerity. She always acknowledges the support of her loving family, especially her husband, Dr Govind N Hoskeri, who has been a driving force behind her success and achievements.

******

Chapter 1

"From Kitchen to Glam: The Pros of Making Your Beauty Goodies"

"Routine hacking starts with ingredients. Everyone has their unique skin quirks. Getting comfortable with ingredient lists is your first step in figuring out what works for you — and what doesn't." — Victoria Fu.

The advantages of using **homemade cosmetics** range from personalization and cost-effectiveness to the assurance of using safe, natural ingredients. Making your moisturizers, face packs, and lip balms in a world saturated with beauty products loaded with chemicals and preservatives empowers you to prioritize health, sustainability, and creativity.

Complete Control Over the Ingredients

- Synthetic chemicals in many commercial products might harm skin health. By choosing to make your cosmetics, you can select high-quality, natural ingredients tailored to your skin type and preferences.
- This customization ensures that your skincare products are free from potentially harmful additives, promoting skin well-being.
- Using safe ingredients in homemade cosmetics addresses concerns related to allergies and sensitivities. Commercial products often include allergens and harsh chemicals that can trigger adverse reactions.
- Making your skincare items enables you to eliminate these potential irritants, fostering a gentler and more nourishing approach to skincare.
- Cost-effectiveness is another added advantage. While some high-end commercial products come with hefty price tags, making your cosmetics at home can be budget-friendly.
- Basic ingredients like coconut oil, honey, aloe vera, saffron, turmeric, almond, and essential oils are often more affordable, making DIY skincare economical. You can select any of these safe ingredients as per your preference, and that suit

your skin type. For example, if you have acne-prone skin, using a dash of licorice powder and a pinch of cinnamon powder along with a pinch of wild turmeric in your face packs is helpful, as these three are antiseptic and anti-bacterial and promote healing effects.

Environmental Sustainability

- The excessive packaging used by commercial manufacturers harms the environment.
- By creating your skincare products at home, you reduce the demand for single-use plastic containers and minimize your carbon footprint.
- By incorporating reusable packaging options, you align your beauty routine with eco-conscious practices.

A Deeper Connection with Self-care

- Engaging in creating your skincare routine transforms it into a mindful and therapeutic experience.
- Choosing different ingredients allows you to discover what works best for your skin, turning skincare into a personalized ritual that caters to your unique needs.

- Homemade cosmetics are creative experiences. Formulating your skincare items empowers you to experiment with textures, scents, and beneficial properties of various ingredients. This creative exploration can be a fulfilling and enjoyable aspect of self-expression, turning your beauty routine into artistry.
- The transparency of homemade cosmetics is a stark departure from the often-confusing ingredient lists on commercial products. Our skin has a rich network of blood vessels underneath, and we have minute pores on the skin, which quickly absorb whatever we apply.
- So, chemical-free applications that are natural, made from what is available in your kitchen, are more skin-safe and rewarding.
- Knowing what goes into your skincare items provides peace of mind and builds confidence in the safety and efficacy of the products you use. This transparency is especially valuable for those with specific skin concerns or conditions who may require a more tailored approach to skincare.

A Back-to-Basics Approach

- Emphasizing the simplicity and purity of natural ingredients aligns with the growing movement towards minimalism and clean beauty.
- It highlights the idea that skincare can be a simple process. The benefits of homemade cosmetics extend beyond personal use. They present an opportunity for small-scale entrepreneurship.
- Many individuals have turned their passion for crafting skincare items into a business, creating and selling handmade products to like-minded consumers.
- It not only provides an avenue for economic empowerment but also contributes to the diversification of the beauty industry.

Conclusion

The benefits of making homemade cosmetics using safe ingredients are diverse and impactful.

From customization and cost-effectiveness to sustainability and creativity, the advantages extend beyond individual skincare to encompass broader environmental and societal considerations. Homemade elixirs encourage a holistic approach to skincare.

Skincare products can foster a deeper connection to the ingredients used and the self-care routine. Mixing ingredients, applying, and taking time for self-pampering can promote well-being and mindfulness.

******

Important Considerations for Skincare

"Good skincare is a lifetime commitment"—Georgia Louise

While homemade face beauty aids offer many benefits, there are essential considerations to keep in mind.

Patch Testing

Before applying any homemade moisturizers and packs to the face, it's advisable to use them on a small portion of the dorsum of your palm and check whether it suits your skin type. It is called a skin patch test.

Hygiene

You must maintain proper hygiene when preparing and storing to prevent bacterial growth. Using clean utensils, containers, and ingredients is crucial.

Shelf Life

Unlike commercial products with preservatives, homemade ones have a **limited shelf life** because of the absence of additives. Preparing smaller batches to ensure freshness and efficacy is always advisable.

Consistency

Achieving the right consistency and texture requires handpicking the ingredients that complement each other in proportion and understanding the balance of the right ingredients to suit one's preferences.

If you follow the steps in this book, you can make and use these fabulous beauty aids with little effort.

If you have any skin condition or are undergoing treatment, **please consult your medical caregiver**.

******

Chapter 2

"In Tune with Your Skin: A Guide to Skin Type Awareness."

"Skin is as unique as we are, and understanding its type is essential for effective skincare."

Introduction

We can classify skin into five types: normal, oily, dry, combination, and sensitive. Identifying your skin type involves assessing factors like oiliness, dryness, and sensitivity. Once you know your skin type, tailored care can help maintain its balance and health, leading to a great complexion.

Your skin, much like a fingerprint, is distinctly individual, and comprehending its unique characteristics is important for a successful skincare regimen. With this knowledge, we can take care to preserve the delicate equilibrium of the skin, ultimately resulting in a radiant and healthy complexion.

Our skin, as diverse as the individuals it graces and its uniqueness, demands a nuanced understanding of effective skincare.

Each skin type comes with its distinct characteristics, forming a roadmap for personalized care. Identification of your specific skin type entails a thoughtful assessment of factors such as oiliness, dryness, and sensitivity.

Normal skin maintains a well-balanced state, neither too oily nor excessively dry. Oily skin produces more sebum, leading to a glossy appearance, while dry skin lacks sufficient moisture, often resulting in flakiness or tightness.

Combination skin, a blend of different types in various areas, presents a unique set of challenges. Sensitive skin is susceptible to irritation, allergies, and reactions, requiring gentle care.

By understanding the intricacies of your skin, you empower yourself to make informed choices in selecting products and adopting practices that maintain its delicate balance and promote overall health.

The personalized approach to skin type lays the foundation for a radiant complexion that reflects the beauty of your individuality.

Skin Types

The five main skin types are normal, oily, dry, combination, and sensitive.

Normal Skin

How do you identify normal skin?

- Normal skin is well-balanced, not too oily nor too dry. It appears clear and smooth.
- It has a healthy complexion.
- Pores on the skin typically remain small, and there is a general balance in oil production.

How to take care?

- Normal skin requires a balanced approach.
- Use a gentle cleanser to remove impurities without stripping natural oils.
- Moisturize regularly to maintain hydration.
- Sunscreen is crucial for protection, and occasional exfoliation helps promote skin renewal.
- Our skin needs hydration to remain healthy. Intake of plenty of water daily keeps the skin healthy.

Oily Skin

How to Identify Oily Skin?

- Excess sebum production characterizes Oily skin.
- It often looks shiny, especially in the T-zone (forehead, nose, and chin).
- Pores may appear enlarged, and individuals with oily skin are prone to acne and blackheads.

How To Take Care of Oily Skin?

- Cleansing is vital to managing excess oil.
- Choose oil-free and non-comedogenic products.
- Use a gentle, hydrating moisturizer to prevent the skin from overcompensating with more oil.
- Regular exfoliation can help unclog pores.
- A clay mask can occasionally absorb excess oil.
- Take care of your diet and avoid fried food and junk food. Have plenty of fruits and vegetables in your diet.

Dry Skin

How to Identify Dry Skin?

- Dry skin lacks moisture, often feeling tight and flaky. It may appear dull, and fine lines can be more noticeable.
- Dry skin often leads to redness and irritation and can feel rough to the touch if proper care is not taken.

How to Take Care of Dry Skin?

- Hydration is key. Use a mild, moisturizing cleanser.
- Apply a rich, nourishing moisturizer regularly, especially after bathing.
- Incorporate hydrating ingredients like hyaluronic acid and avoid harsh drying products.
- Exfoliate gently to remove dead skin cells.
- Drink plenty of water. Increase intake of fluids like soups, buttermilk, and fruit juices.
- Use chickpea flour to cleanse your skin. It keeps the skin nourished and soft.

Combination Skin

How to Identify Combination Skin?

- When we have different skin types on different parts of the face or body, it is called combination skin.

- For example, the T-zone is often oily, while the cheeks may be normal or dry. Balancing both can be challenging.

How to Take Care of Combination Skin?

- Use a gentle, balanced cleanser.

- Moisturize according to the needs of different areas – lightweight for oily zones and richer for dry areas.

- Spot-treat oily areas and provide extra hydration where needed.

- Regular exfoliation can maintain overall skin health.

Sensitive or Reactive Skin

How do you know if your skin is reactive?

- If you have sensitive skin, then it is prone to redness, itching, and irritation.
- It may react to certain products, weather, or environmental factors.
- Sensitive skin can be any type—normal, oily, dry, or combination.

How to Take Care of Sensitive Skin?

- Use fragrance-free and hypoallergenic products.
- Before trying out anything new on your skin, apply it to a small area on your hand and wait and watch. Only if it suits you, try it on your face, neck, or all over your body.
- Use a gentle cleanser and a moisturizer with soothing ingredients like chamomile or aloe vera.
- Sun protection is crucial and avoids harsh chemicals or excessive exfoliation.

Understanding your skin type goes beyond these categories—it involves recognizing specific concerns like acne-prone, mature, or pigmentation-prone skin.

Here's a detailed guide on caring for each skin type:

Skincare Tips

Normal Skin Care

- **Cleansing:** Use a mild, hydrating cleanser morning and night.

- **Moisturizing:** Apply a balanced moisturizer to maintain hydration.

- **Sunscreen:** Protect your skin with a broad-spectrum SPF of at least 30.

- **Exfoliation:** Once or twice a week with a gentle exfoliant to promote cell turnover.

Oily Skin Care

- **Cleansing:** Use a foaming or gel cleanser to control oil.

- **Moisturizing**: Choose an oil-free, non-comedogenic moisturizer.

- **Sunscreen**: Use a lightweight, oil-free SPF.

- **Exfoliation**: 2-3 times a week with a salicylic acid or gentle scrub.

Dry Skin Care

• **Cleansing:** Use a creamy, hydrating cleanser.

• **Moisturizing**: Apply a rich, emollient moisturizer regularly.

• **Sunscreen:** Choose a moisturizing SPF to protect against UV rays.

• **Exfoliation:** 1-2 times a week with a mild exfoliant to avoid over-drying.

Combination Skin Care

• **Cleansing:** Use a balanced, gentle cleanser.

• **Moisturizing:** Tailor your moisturizer to different areas—lightweight for oily zones, richer for dry.

• **Sunscreen**: Go for a broad-spectrum SPF suitable for your skin's needs.

• **Exfoliation:** focus on maintaining balance; adjust frequency as needed.

Sensitive Skin Care

- **Cleansing:** Use a mild, fragrance-free cleanser.

- **Moisturizing:** Choose a hypoallergenic, soothing moisturizer.

- **Sunscreen:** Use a mineral sunscreen with gentle ingredients.

- **Exfoliation:** Be cautious; opt for enzymatic or gentle exfoliants sparingly.

Beyond daily care, lifestyle factors contribute to skin health. Stay hydrated, maintain a balanced diet rich in antioxidants, and manage stress levels. Regular professional skincare consultations can provide personalized advice.

Last, adapt your skincare routine to the seasons–your skin's needs may change with weather variations. Listen to your skin, adjust your routine, and enjoy the journey to healthy, radiant skin.

******

Chapter 3:
Why do Moisturizers Matter for Our Skin?

Introduction

Skin is the largest organ of our body, and maintaining its health is essential for overall well-being. One of the key elements in a skincare routine that contributes significantly to skin health is the use of moisturizers that help hydrate and nourish the skin, playing a crucial role in promoting a radiant and youthful complexion.

A radiant and healthy skin appearance is crucial, as any imperfections can lead to a decline in self-esteem. Moisturizers play a significant role in addressing fine lines, smoothing the skin, ensuring proper hydration, and enhancing social life, psychological well-being, and overall quality of life. Whether dealing with normal skin or dermatoses exhibiting dry skin symptoms, both can derive optimal advantages from the use of moisturizers.

The manifestation of skin dryness involves noticeable and tactile alterations in the skin, accompanied by changes in its sensory components, presenting as symptoms of dry skin. These symptoms encompass sensations of dryness and various discomforts, including tightness, pain, itching, stinging, and tingling.

Moisturizers prove highly effective in addressing the underlying dermatoses causing dry skin, disrupting the cycle of dryness while maintaining the smoothness of the skin. Moisturizers offer multiple benefits beyond mere skin moisturization.

1. Hydration Helps Moisture Retention

The primary function of moisturizers is to hydrate the skin. Our skin constantly loses moisture because of various factors, such as environmental conditions, aging, and daily activities. Moisturizers contain ingredients like humectants that gather and keep moisture from the surrounding environment, helping to keep the skin hydrated, emollients that soften and smooth the skin, improving its texture and flexibility, and occlusive that form a protective barrier on the skin's surface, preventing moisture loss and enhancing hydration.

Together, these components contribute to a comprehensive approach to skincare, addressing moisture retention, texture improvement, and barrier protection. Well-hydrated skin not only feels softer but also looks healthier and more vibrant.

2. Preventing Dryness and Flakiness

Dry, flaky skin not only causes discomfort but can also lead to various skin issues. Moisturizers act as a barrier, preventing the skin from becoming excessively dry. By providing a protective layer, they help reduce dryness and flakiness, promoting a smoother and more even skin texture.

3. Soothing Irritation and Redness

Sensitive skin can experience irritation and redness because of environmental factors, allergies, or harsh skincare products. Moisturizers made of aloe vera, chamomile, or calendula can soothe the skin, bring down redness, and ease discomfort, making them useful for individuals with reactive skin.

4. Anti-Aging Benefits

As we age, the skin's ability to retain moisture diminishes, leading to the development of fine lines and wrinkles. Moisturizers with anti-aging properties, such as collagen-boosting peptides and antioxidants, can help reduce the appearance of wrinkles and promote a more youthful complexion. Regular use of moisturizers can contribute to the long-term health and vitality of the skin.

5. Enhancing Elasticity of Skin

Skin becomes less elastic as we age. Moisturizers play a role in maintaining and enhancing skin elasticity by keeping the skin well-hydrated and supple. This elasticity not only contributes to a more youthful appearance but also helps the skin withstand various external stressors.

Balancing Oil Production

Contrary to a common misconception, even individuals with oily skin can benefit from using moisturizers. In fact, the right moisturizer can help balance oil production. Dehydrated skin can compensate by producing more oil, which leads to increased breakouts. By providing adequate hydration, moisturizers can prevent the skin from overproducing oil, promoting a healthier complexion.

6. Improving Skin Tone and Texture

Regular use of moisturizers can contribute to an improvement in overall skin tone and texture. Some moisturizers help in exfoliation by removing dead skin cells and making it a smoother, more radiant complexion.

7. Protection Against Environmental Stressors

When the skin gets exposed to pollution, UV radiation, and harsh weather, moisturizers with added sun protection (SPF) help to protect against the harmful effects of harsh sun rays, reducing the risk of premature aging and skin damage.

Conclusion

The benefits of using moisturizers for our skin are diverse and significant. From maintaining hydration and preventing dryness to addressing specific skin concerns like irritation and aging, a well-formulated moisturizer is a valuable addition to any skincare routine. By knowing the actual needs of our skin and choosing the right moisturizer, we can nurture and protect our skin, promoting a healthy and radiant complexion for years to come.

******

How do Moisturizers Work?

The skin serves as a protective barrier, shielding underlying tissues from desiccation, infection, mechanical stress, and chemical irritation. A compromised function results in an escalating trans-epidermal water loss, particularly seen in various forms of dermatitis.

The intricate process involves water from deeper epidermal layers ascending to hydrate stratum corneum cells, only to be lost through evaporation. Maintaining adequate epidermal water content is crucial to prevent skin dryness and sustain elasticity.

The stratum corneum, resembling a bricks-and-mortar model, relies on the integrity of intercellular lipids—such as ceramide, cholesterol, and fatty acids—to form bilayers, safeguarding against water barrier damage and subsequent dry skin.

The stratum corneum's structure plays a pivotal role in regulating skin water flux, retention, and overall moisturization. Four essential processes govern its formation and function: corneocyte, stratum corneum lipid, natural moisturizing factor, and desquamation. Corneocytes act as a physical barrier, contributing to elasticity when adequately hydrated.

The lipid bilayers serve as a moisture barrier, simultaneously preventing chemical entry and enabling the absorption of topically applied substances. External humidity influences the natural moisturizing factor, which comprises hygroscopic molecules and sustains corneocyte hydration. Desquamation involves the degradation of a process less efficient in a low-moisture stratum corneum, leading to the appearance of dry skin signs.

Moisturizers play a pivotal role in skin barrier repair, preserving skin integrity, and enhancing appearance through their roles as humectants, emollients, and occlusive.

By directly providing water, reducing trans-epidermal water loss, covering fissures, and creating a protective film, moisturizers improve hydration and increase stratum corneum water content. They smooth the skin surface, filling spaces between desquamated skin flakes and restoring the ability of intercellular lipid bilayers to absorb, retain, and redistribute water.

This dynamic process alters skin mechanics, facilitating the degradation, preventing corneocyte accumulation, and promoting skin continuity. Research by Loden emphasizes that skincare products don't merely stay on the skin's surface but penetrate it to influence its structure and function actively.

Conclusion

For maintaining healthy and radiant skin, moisturizers play an important role in our skincare routine, offering many benefits that extend beyond mere cosmetic appeal. Moisturizers are not just about achieving a dewy complexion but are essential for the overall health and wellbeing of our skin by combating dryness.

We constantly expose our skin to external factors like pollution and harsh sun rays that can take away its natural moisture. Harsh weather, pollution, and even daily cleansing routines can leave the skin dehydrated and prone to dehydration. Moisturizers act as a barrier, sealing in moisture and preventing water loss. By replenishing the skin's hydration levels, moisturizers fortify its natural defenses against external aggressors.

Moisturizers contribute significantly to maintaining the skin's elasticity and suppleness. As we age, the skin undergoes a natural process of losing collagen and elastin proteins responsible for its firmness and flexibility. Regular application of moisturizers helps in mitigating this loss, promoting a more youthful appearance. The hydrating ingredients in moisturizers, such as glycerine, work to plump the skin, reducing the visibility of fine lines and wrinkles. Moisturizers have become a reliable ally in the battle against premature aging, allowing us to embrace the aging process with grace.

Dry and cracked skin not only looks unattractive but can also become a breeding ground for various skin issues. Moisturizers act as a preventive measure against conditions like eczema and dermatitis by maintaining the skin's integrity. Moisturizers shield the skin from irritants and allergens, reducing the risk of inflammation and discomfort.

Whether you have oily, dry, sensitive, or combination skin, there is a moisturizer you can tailor to meet your unique needs. This inclusivity ensures individuals can address their specific skin issues, promoting a personalized approach to skincare. From lightweight gel-based formulations for oily skin to rich creams for intense hydration, DIY moisturizers offer options for everyone.

Regular use of moisturizers helps promote a positive skincare routine. Applying moisturizer is a ritual that extends beyond the physical benefits; it is an act of self-care. The tactile sensation of massaging moisturizer into the skin improves blood circulation and provides a moment of tranquillity in our hectic lives.

This simple yet meaningful practice fosters a connection with oneself, encouraging mindfulness and nurturing a positive relationship with one's body.

In a nutshell, the significance of moisturizers for our skin transcends the surface, diving deep into our focus on health, confidence, and self-care. These unassuming products wield the power to protect, rejuvenate, and uplift our skin, allowing it to thrive amidst the challenges of modern living.

As we embrace the holistic approach to skincare, let moisturizers take center stage in our daily routines, guiding us towards not just beautiful skin but skin that is resilient, vibrant, and a reflection of our overall well-being.

******

Chapter 4: Unveiling the Secrets of Natural Moisturizers

"Take care of your skin, and your confidence will take care of itself." — Amit Kalantri.

Embracing the art of making your skincare moisturizers is a holistic approach that prioritizes well-being, self-expression, and a conscious connection to the beauty that nature provides.

Herbal Moisturizers for Normal Skin Type

1. Aloe Vera and Coconut Oil

Ingredients required

- five tablespoons of aloe vera gel
- 2 ½ tablespoons of coconut oil
- one teaspoon of vitamin E oil (or contents of 6 capsules of Vitamin E)

Preparation and Use

- Combine aloe vera gel, coconut oil, and vitamin E oil in a clean glass bowl.
- Mix thoroughly until smooth consistency.
- Fill a clean, airtight container with the mixture. Apply a small amount to your face and body for a hydrating and soothing effect.

2. Cocoa Butter and Shea Butter Bliss

Ingredients required

- Two tablespoons of cocoa butter
- Two tablespoons shea butter
- 1 tablespoon jojoba oil
- One teaspoon of almond oil or coconut oil

Preparation and Use

- Melt shea and cocoa butter in a double boiler until fully melted.
- Let the mixture cool slightly, then add jojoba oil.
- Stir well and let it solidify slightly.
- Whip the mixture with a hand mixer until fluffy.
- Store in a jar and apply as needed.

3. Honey and Almond Oil Delight

Ingredients required

- six tablespoons of almond oil
- two tablespoons of honey
- one tablespoon beeswax (optional for thicker consistency)

Preparation and Use

- In a heat-safe container, combine almond oil and honey.
- If using beeswax, melt it with the mixture using a double boiler.
- Thoroughly combine the ingredients by stirring well.
- Allow the mixture to cool, and transfer it to a jar.
- Apply this nourishing moisturizer to keep your skin supple and moisturized.

4. Green Tea and Olive Oil Hydration

Ingredients required

- 50 ml of brewed and cooled green tea.
- Two tablespoons of olive oil.
- One tablespoon of aloe vera gel.

Preparation and Use

- Mix cooled green tea, olive oil, and aloe vera gel in a bowl.
- Stir until well combined.
- Fill the container with the mixture and store it in the refrigerator.
- Use this refreshing moisturizer for a burst of hydration on your normal skin.

5. Rosewater and Glycerine Elegance

Ingredients required

- 50 ml of rosewater
- two tablespoons of glycerine
- 1 tablespoon jojoba oil

Preparation and Use

- Combine rosewater, glycerine, and jojoba oil in a mixing bowl.
- Mix thoroughly until well combined.
- Pour the mixture into a bottle with a spray nozzle for easy application.
- Spray on your face and body for a light, fragrant, moisturizing experience.

6. Avocado and Yogurt Soothing Cream

Ingredients required

- Five tablespoons of ripe avocado.
- Two tablespoons of plain yogurt.
- One tablespoon olive oil.
- Six drops of rosemary essential oil (optional).

Preparation and Use

- Mash the ripe avocado in a bowl until smooth.
- Add yogurt and olive oil, then mix well.
- Apply this creamy mixture to your skin for a nourishing and hydrating effect.
- Rinse off after 15-20 minutes for soft and supple skin.

Remember to perform a patch test before using any new homemade moisturizer to ensure compatibility with your skin. These recipes offer a range of textures and scents, allowing you to choose the one that best suits your preferences while providing effective hydration for normal skin.

Herbal Moisturizers for Dry Skin

1. Shea Butter and Coconut Oil Bliss

Ingredients required

- A measurement of two tablespoons of shea butter
- Measure two tablespoons of cocoa butter
- Two tablespoons of coconut oil
- One tablespoon of sweet almond oil

Preparation and Use

- Melt coconut oil along with shea butter in a double boiler until fully melted.
- Add sweet almond oil and stir well.
- Allow the mixture to cool, then whip it until fluffy.
- Transfer to a jar and apply generously for deep moisturization.
- Shelf Life: Approximately six months.
- Storage: Store in a cool, dark place.

2. Oatmeal and Honey Soothing Cream

Ingredients required

Six tablespoons of oatmeal (ground into a fine powder)

Two tablespoons honey

Five tablespoons of

Preparation and Use

- Mix oatmeal, honey, and yogurt until you achieve a smooth consistency.
- Apply the mixture to your skin and leave it on for 15-20 minutes.
- Rinse off with warm water.

Shelf Life: Use immediately or refrigerate for up to 1 week.

Storage: Keep refrigerated if not used immediately.

3. **Avocado and Olive Oil Nourishing Cream for dry Skin**

Ingredients required

- Four tablespoons of ripe avocado paste
- Two tablespoons of olive oil
- One tablespoon of argan oil

Preparation and Use

- Mash the ripe avocado until smooth.
- Add olive oil and argan oil and mix well.
- Apply to dry areas for intense hydration.

Shelf Life: Use within 2-3 days if kept refrigerated.

Storage: Refrigerate if not used immediately.

4. Cocoa Butter and Almond Oil Elegance

Ingredients required

- Two tablespoons of cocoa butter
- Two tablespoons of almond oil
- 1 tablespoon jojoba oil
- Six drops of rosemary essential oil

Preparation and Use

- Warm cocoa butter in a double boiler, then add almond oil and jojoba oil.
- Stir well and let it cool.
- Whip the mixture until fluffy.
- Apply as needed for a luxurious moisturizing experience.

• Shelf Life: Approximately 6-8 months.

• Storage: Keep in a cool, dark place.

5. Coconut Milk and almond Oil Moisture Boost

Ingredients required

- 50 ml of coconut milk
- Two tablespoons of almond oil
- One tablespoon of vitamin E oil

Preparation and Use

- Mix coconut milk, olive oil, and vitamin E oil in a bowl.
- Stir well until thoroughly combined.
- Apply to dry skin for a nourishing and rejuvenating effect.

• Shelf Life: Approximately 1-2 weeks if kept refrigerated.

• Storage: Refrigerate and use within the specified time frame.

6. Honey and Beeswax Protective Cream

Ingredients required

- Two tablespoons honey
- Two tablespoons beeswax
- Three tablespoons olive oil

Preparation and Use

- Melt beeswax in a double boiler, then add honey and olive oil.
- Stir until well combined, then let it cool.
- Apply as needed for a protective barrier against dryness.

• Shelf Life: Approximately 3-4 months.

• Storage: Keep in a cool, dark place.

Herbal Moisturizers for Oily Skin

1. **Tea Tree and Aloe Vera Mattifying Moisturizer**

Ingredients required

- Six tablespoons of aloe vera gel
- 5-7 drops of tea tree oil or any other essential oil of your choice
- One tablespoon of witch hazel

Preparation and Use

- Mix aloe vera gel, tea tree oil, and witch hazel in a bowl.
- Thoroughly combine the ingredients by stirring them well.
- Transfer the mixture to a bottle for easy application.
- Apply to oily skin for a lightweight and impressive effect.

• Shelf Life: Approximately 1-2 months.

• Storage: Keep in a cool, dark place.

2. Cucumber and Mint Refreshing Gel

Ingredients Required

- 1/2 cucumber (blended).
- One tablespoon of mint leaves (finely chopped).
- Two tablespoons of aloe vera gel.

Preparation and Use

- Blend cucumber and finely chop mint leaves.
- Mix the cucumber puree, mint leaves, and aloe vera gel.
- Apply the gel to your face for a refreshing and hydrating sensation.

• Shelf Life: Use immediately or refrigerate for up to 3 days.

• Storage: Refrigerate if not used immediately.

3. Jojoba Oil and Green Tea Moisture Control

Ingredients required

- Two tablespoons of jojoba oil.
- 50 ml of brewed green tea (cooled).
- One tablespoon of aloe vera gel.

Preparation and Use

- Combine jojoba oil, green tea, and aloe vera gel in a bowl.
- Mix well until the ingredients form a lightweight moisturizer.
- Store in a clean container and refrigerate.
- Apply to oily skin for balanced hydration.

• Shelf Life: Approximately two months.

• Storage: Keep in a cool, dark place.

4. **Rosewater and Lavender Oil Hydrating Mist**

Ingredients required

- 50 ml of rosewater
- 5-7 drops of lavender essential oil
- One tablespoon glycerine

Preparation and Use

- Mix rosewater, lavender oil, and glycerine in a bottle.
- Shake well before use and spray on your face for a light, hydrating mist.

• Shelf Life: Approximately 2-3 months.

• Storage: Keep in a cool, dark place.

5. Charcoal and Clay Detoxifying Moisturizer

Ingredients required

- One tablespoon of activated charcoal powder
- Two tablespoons bentonite clay
- 1/4 cup water

Preparation and Use

- Mix activated charcoal powder, bentonite clay, and water in a bowl.
- Keep stirring until you form a smooth paste.
- Apply a thin layer to your face for a detoxifying and oil-absorbing effect.
- Wash it off after 5-10 minutes.

• Shelf Life: Use immediately or refrigerate for up to 1 week.

• Storage: Refrigerate if not used immediately.

6. Lemon and Yogurt Lotion

Ingredients required

Two tablespoons of unsweetened yogurt

One tablespoon of fresh lemon juice

A pinch of wild turmeric

Preparation and Use

- Mix yogurt, lemon juice, turmeric, and aloe vera gel until well combined.
- Apply the mixture to your face for a brightening effect.

• Shelf Life: Use immediately or refrigerate for up to 3 days.

• Storage: Refrigerate if not used immediately.

Adjust ingredient quantities based on your preferences and skin sensitivity. Always perform patch tests, especially with essential oils, to ensure compatibility with your skin. These recipes cater to oily skin, providing hydration without adding excess oil.

Moisturizers for Combination Skin

1. Shea Butter and Almond Oil

Ingredients Required

- Four tablespoons of shea butter
- Two tablespoons of almond oil
- Few drops of any essential oil of your preference (optional, for fragrance.

Preparation and Use

- In a double boiler, melt the shea butter and add almond oil.
- Let the mixture cool slightly, then add the essential oil if using, and mix well.
- Transfer the mixture to a clean, airtight container.
- To use, take a small amount and gently massage it onto your face and body after cleansing.
- Use daily, especially after showering or washing your face.

2. Aloe Vera and Jojoba Oil

Ingredients Required

- Four tablespoons of aloe vera gel.
- 1 tablespoon jojoba oil.
- Fifteen drops of vitamin E oil; if you don't have this oil, then cut six capsules of vitamin E and use. Vitamin E nourishes the skin, and it also is a natural preservative.

Preparation and Use

- In a bowl, combine the aloe vera gel and jojoba oil.
- If using, add the vitamin E oil and mix thoroughly.
- Store the mixture in a clean, airtight container.
- Apply a small amount of the moisturizer to your face and body after cleansing.
- Gently massage until absorbed. Use daily, morning and night. It gives wonderful results.

3. Olive Oil and Beeswax

Ingredients Required

- Four tablespoons of olive oil
- One tablespoon grated beeswax
- A few drops of essential oil, if you like

Preparation and Use

- In a double boiler, melt the grated beeswax and olive oil until fully combined.
- Let the mixture cool, and then add the essential oil.
- Store the mixture in a clean container.
- Let it solidify **at room temperature**.
- Scoop out a small amount and warm it between your fingers before applying it to your skin.
- Massage gently until absorbed. Use as needed.

4. Cocoa Butter and Almond Oil

Ingredients Required

Five tablespoons of cocoa butter

Two tablespoons of almond oil

5-10 drops of rose essential oil (optional for fragrance)

Preparation and Use

- Warm the cocoa butter in a double boiler.
- Once melted, add the almond oil and rose essential oil (if using).
- Mix properly and let the mixture cool.
- Transfer to a clean, airtight container.
- Let it **solidify at room temperature.**
- Apply a small amount to your skin and massage until absorbed. Use daily.

5. Yogurt and Honey

Ingredients Required

- Four tablespoons of full-fat plain yogurt
- One tablespoon of honey
- One teaspoon of the almond oil, olive oil, or sesame oil

Preparation and Use

- In a bowl, mix the plain yogurt, honey, and olive or sesame oil until well combined.
- Cleanse your face and pat it dry.
- Apply the mixture to your face and neck.
- Leave it on for about ten minutes.
- Rinse off with lukewarm water and pat your skin dry.

6   Avocado and Almond Oil

Ingredients Required

- Four tablespoons of ripe avocado pulp
- One tablespoon of almond oil
- 5-6 drops of cinnamon oil (optional) or one teaspoon of cinnamon powder

Preparation and Use

- Cut the ripe avocado in half and scoop out the flesh.
- Mash the avocado until smooth.
- Mix in the almond oil to create a consistent mixture.
- Cinnamon oil or cinnamon powder helps control acne.
- Cleanse your face and pat it dry.
- Apply the avocado and almond oil mixture to your face and neck.
- Leave it on for about ten minutes.
- Rinse off with lukewarm water and pat your skin dry.

Herbal Moisturizers for Sensitive Skin

1. Green Tea and Rosehip Oil

Ingredients Required

- 50 ml of brewed and cooled green tea
- One tablespoon of rosehip oil
- One teaspoon of vegetable glycerine (optional for added hydration
- Or one tablespoon of aloe vera gel

Preparation and Use

- Brew 50 ml of green tea and let it cool completely.
- Mix the brewed green tea and rosehip oil.
- If using, add the vegetable glycerine or aloe vera and mix.
- Store the mixture in a clean, airtight container.
- Apply a small amount to your face and neck after cleansing.
- Gently massage until absorbed. Use daily for better results.

2. Coconut Milk and Lavender

Ingredients Required

- Five tablespoons of coconut milk
- One tablespoon of sweet almond oil
- 5-10 drops of lavender essential oil

Preparation and use

- Mix the coconut milk and sweet almond oil in a bowl.
- Add the lavender essential oil and stir well to combine.
- Store the mixture in a clean, airtight container.
- Apply a small amount to your skin after cleansing.
- Massage with fingertips until absorbed.

3. Cucumber and Mint

Ingredients Required

- Five tablespoons of clear cucumber juice
- One tablespoon of grapeseed oil or sesame oil
- 5-10 drops of peppermint essential oil

Preparation and Use

- Blend a cucumber to extract its juice. Strain the juice to remove any residue.
- Mix the cucumber juice and grapeseed oil.
- Add the sesame or peppermint essential oil and mix well.
- Store the mixture in a clean, airtight container.
- Apply to your skin after cleansing.
- Massage until absorbed. Use daily.

4. **Honey and Almond Butter**

Ingredients Required

- Two tablespoons of almond butter
- One tablespoon honey
- One teaspoon of jojoba oil

Preparation and Use

- Mix the almond butter, honey, and jojoba oil well until you have a smooth consistency.
- Cleanse your face and pat it dry.
- Apply a small amount of the mixture to your face and neck.
- Gently massage until absorbed. Use daily.

5. Papaya and Coconut Cream

Ingredients Required

- Five tablespoons of mashed and strained ripe papaya
- Two tablespoons of coconut cream
- One teaspoon of vitamin E oil (oil from 6 to 7 capsules of vitamin E)

Preparation and Use

- Mash the ripe papaya until it's smooth.
- Mix in the coconut cream and vitamin E oil.
- Cleanse your face and pat it dry.
- Apply the mixture to your skin.
- Massage until absorbed. Use it regularly.

6. Banana Cocoa Powder Delight

Ingredients Required

- One ripe banana
- One tablespoon of cocoa powder
- 1,5 teaspoon of coconut oil

Preparation and Use

- Mash the ripe banana until smooth.
- Mix in the cocoa powder and coconut oil.
- Cleanse your face and pat it dry.
- Apply a small amount of the mixture to your face and neck.
- Leave it on for about twelve minutes.
- Rinse off with lukewarm water and pat your skin dry.

7. **Greek Yogurt and Honey**

Ingredients Required

- Five tablespoons of Greek yogurt
- One tablespoon of honey
- One teaspoon of olive oil

Preparation and Use

- Mix the Greek yogurt, honey, and olive oil until smooth.
- Cleanse your face and wipe it dry.
- Apply it evenly to your face and neck.
- Leave it on for about ten minutes.
- Rinse off with water at room temperature.

8. Green Tea and Aloe Vera Gel

Ingredients Required

- 50 ml of brewed and cooled green tea.
- Two tablespoons of aloe vera gel.

Preparation and Use

- Mix green tea and aloe vera gel, and apply.
- Green tea is rich in antioxidants, and aloe vera soothes the skin.

Chapter 5:
Homemade Packs for a Radiant Skin

Introduction

Face packs are a part of the skincare regime. Homemade Face Packs have gained popularity for several reasons. First, they offer a more personalized approach to skincare, allowing individuals to choose ingredients based on their specific skin needs.

Common ingredients found in homemade face packs include natural substances like honey, yogurt, sugar, rice, aloe vera, and fruits. These ingredients, with their potential to nourish, hydrate, and rejuvenate the skin, are good for the skin.

One key benefit of using homemade face packs is the avoidance of harmful chemicals often present in commercially produced skincare products. Many store-bought packs contain preservatives, artificial fragrances, and other additives that may not be suitable for all skin types. By creating Packs at home, individuals can have better control over the ingredients they apply to their faces, minimizing the risk of adverse reactions.

Homemade Face Packs Can Contribute to a Radiant Complexion.

Hydration and Moisturization

Ingredients like honey and yogurt have moisturizing properties. They help replenish the skin's moisture content, preventing dryness and promoting a soft texture. Proper hydration is crucial for a glowing complexion and skin's elasticity to reduce the appearance of fine lines.

Nutrient Boost

Fruits like strawberries, bananas, and papayas are rich in vitamins and antioxidants. These nutrients help nourish the skin, protect it from environmental factors, and promote a youthful glow. Vitamins like C and E are good for their skin-brightening and combating free radicals.

Exfoliation

Homemade face packs often contain natural exfoliants like oatmeal, rice flour, or finely ground almonds. These ingredients help remove dead skin cells, unclog pores, and promote cell turnover. Regular exfoliation is crucial for achieving a brighter complexion by revealing fresh, healthy skin underneath.

Anti-Inflammatory Effects

Ingredients such as aloe vera, turmeric, and chamomile possess anti-inflammatory properties, which can calm skin irritation and reduce redness. It is beneficial for individuals with sensitive or acne-prone skin, as inflammation can contribute to a dull complexion.

Stress Reduction

The process of applying a homemade face pack can be a therapeutic and stress-relieving activity. Stress is a known contributor to skin issues, and taking the time for self-care can positively affect both mental well-being and skin health.

Homemade face packs are powerful tools for achieving a radiant and healthy complexion. By incorporating natural and nourishing ingredients into these packs, individuals can customize their skincare routine, steering clear of harsh chemicals and embracing the beauty-enhancing benefits of nature.

Please note that everyone's skin is different, and it is important to try on a small portion of your skin before applying any homemade products to your face to ensure you're not allergic to any of the ingredients. If you experience any irritation or adverse reactions, discontinue use immediately.

Creating homemade skincare products can be a creative and cost-effective activity. Here are some exceptional homemade face packs using fruits and other easily available ingredients, along with detailed steps for each Pack.

Guidelines for Using Face Packs

The frequency of using face packs depends on the specific type of pack and your skin's needs. Here are some general guidelines,

Deep Cleansing Packs

- Use 1-2 times a week for oily or acne-prone skin.
- Use every two weeks for normal or combination skin.

Exfoliating Packs

- 1-2 times a week for most skin types.
- Reduce frequency if you have sensitive or dry skin.

Hydrating and Moisturizing Packs

- 1-2 times a week for dry skin.
- Use as needed for normal or combination skin.

Skin Brightening Packs

- 1-2 times a week for those targeting hyperpigmentation.
- Once every two weeks for maintenance.

Calming and Soothing Packs

- Apply as needed for sensitive skin.
- Use once or twice a week for a calming effect.

Anti-Aging Packs

- 1-2 times a week for mature skin.
- Once a week for prevention in younger age groups.

Acne Control Packs

- 2-3 times a week for acne-prone skin.
- Adjust the frequency based on skin response.

Some Useful Tips for Using Any Face Pack

Patch Test

Always apply a face pack on a small area of skin to ensure you don't have an adverse reaction.

Cleanse Before Application

- Cleanse your face before applying a face pack to remove any makeup, dirt, or impurities for better absorption.
- Raw milk is the best cleanser for your face and neck.

Even Application

Apply the face pack evenly, avoiding the eye area and lips.

Avoid Overuse

- Using face packs too frequently can lead to over-exfoliation or dryness.
- Follow the recommended frequency for the specific type of pack.

Relax Your Body and Mind

- While the face pack is on, relax. Lie down, close your eyes, and enjoy a few minutes of tranquillity.

Follow with Moisturizer

- After rinsing off the face pack, apply a homemade moisturizer of your choice to lock in hydration and maintain skin balance.

Sunscreen Application

- If you use face packs with exfoliating or brightening properties, always follow up with sunscreen during the day to protect your skin from UV rays.

Rotate Different Types

- If you use multiple face packs targeting different concerns, consider rotating them to address various skincare needs.
- Incorporating face packs into your skincare routine can take care of the overall health and appearance of your skin.
- By selecting packs tailored to your skin type, you can enjoy the benefits of a spa-like treatment at home while addressing specific skincare needs.

Chapter 6:

Let's Get into Action! DIY Face Packs.

1. Rice pack

Achieve youthful and radiant skin with a Korean Face Pack that brightens and fights aging.

Required ingredients

- Six tablespoons of raw white or brown rice. Water.
- One tablespoon of coconut oil.

Preparation

- Wash the rice and add the washed rice in a pan.
- Add two cups of water and cook on low flame.
- Blend the cooked rice to a smooth, thick paste.
- Add one tablespoon of coconut oil or almond oil and mix it well. Store it in a clean jar and store it in a cool, dry place or a refrigerator. We can store it for a week.

Use

Apply it on your face and neck, wait for at least 30 minutes, and then wash your face with cool water. Pat dry and apply your moisturizer. Rice increases collagen in the skin, which keeps the skin supple and prevents wrinkles.

2. Strawberry and Yogurt Brightening Pack

Ingredients Needed

- 3-4 ripe strawberries.
- One tablespoon of plain yogurt.
- Half a teaspoon of honey.

Preparation and Use

- Mash strawberries to a smooth paste.
- Mix them with yogurt and honey.
- Apply the pack to your face and neck.
- Leave it on for 10 -15 minutes.
- Rinse with lukewarm water. Strawberries contain vitamin C for a brightening effect.

Advantage

Yogurt nourishes the skin, and honey has a soothing effect.

3. Papaya and Honey Exfoliating Pack

Ingredients Needed

- Three tablespoons of mashed ripe papaya
- One tablespoon of honey

Preparation and Use

- Mix papaya and honey to a smooth paste.
- Apply the mixture to your face, avoiding the eye area.
- Gently massage in circular motions for 2-3 minutes.
- Leave it on for another 5 to 7 minutes.
- Rinse with cool water.

4. Banana and Avocado Hydrating Pack

Ingredients Needed

- Three teaspoons of ripe banana pulp
- Two teaspoons of ripe avocado pulp
- One teaspoon honey

Preparation and Use

- Mash banana and avocado, then mix in honey.
- Apply the Pack evenly and leave it on for 7 to 10 minutes.
- Rinse with lukewarm water.

5. Cucumber and Aloe Vera Soothing Pack

Ingredients Needed

- Three tablespoons of cucumber (peeled and blended)
- Two tablespoons of aloe vera gel (fresh from the leaves or bought from the store)
- Half a teaspoon of coconut or almond oil.

Preparation and Use

- Mix blended cucumber with aloe vera gel.
- Apply to your face and leave it on for 15-20 minutes.
- Rinse with cool water.

6. Orange and Yogurt Exfoliating Pack

Ingredients Needed

- Three tablespoons of orange juice
- One tablespoon of plain yogurt
- One tablespoon of finely ground oats

Preparation and Use

- Mix orange juice, yogurt, and oat flour to form a paste.
- Apply to your face, avoiding the eye area.
- Leave it on for 15 minutes.
- Gently scrub in circular motions before rinsing.

7. Kiwi and Honey Vitamin C Pack

Ingredients Needed

- Three tablespoons of ripe kiwi pulp.
- One tablespoon of honey.
- One teaspoon of almond oil or olive oil.

Preparation and Use

- Mash kiwi and mix with honey and oil
- Please apply it to your face and leave it on for 7 to 10 minutes
- Rinse with cool water

8. Tomato and Lemon Acne-Fighting Pack

Ingredients Needed

- Pulp of one small ripe tomato.
- One teaspoon of lemon juice.
- A pinch of turmeric powder.

Preparation and Use

- Mix blended tomato with lemon juice and turmeric powder.
- Apply to your face, concentrating on areas with acne.
- Leave it on for 6-12 minutes.
- Rinse with cool water.

9. Pineapple and Coconut Oil Radiance Pack

Ingredients Needed

- Three tablespoons of fresh pineapple paste (blended).
- One teaspoon of coconut oil.
- Half a teaspoon of gingelly oil.

Preparation and Use

- Mix blended pineapple with coconut and gingelly oil
- Apply to your face and leave it on for 7 to 10 minutes
- Rinse with lukewarm water

10. Grape and Oatmeal Anti-Aging Pack

Ingredients:

- Three tablespoons of mashed grapes, with seeds removed.
- One tablespoon of oatmeal powder.
- One teaspoon of aloe vera gel.
- Half a teaspoon of edible gum powder, available in Indian stores, is called gond or dink.

Preparation and Use

- Mix mashed grapes with oatmeal powder, aloe vera gel, and powdered gum crystals.
- Let the mixture sit for 3-4 minutes.
- Apply to your face and leave it on for 15-20 minutes.
- Rinse with cool water.

11. Mango and Honey Nourishing Pack

Ingredients Needed

- Three tablespoons of mashed ripe mango (pulp).
- One tablespoon of honey.
- Half a tablespoon of cooked and mashed rice or rice powder.

Preparation and Use

- Mix mango, rice, and honey.
- Apply to your face and leave it on for 10-12 minutes.
- Rinse with lukewarm water.

12. Watermelon and Mint Cooling Pack

Ingredients Needed

¼ cup blended watermelon, a handful of fresh mint leaves (finely chopped)

Mix blended watermelon with chopped mint leaves. Apply to your face and leave it on for 15-20 minutes. Rinse with cool water.

13. Apricot and Almond Oil Exfoliating Pack

Ingredients Needed

- Two ripe apricots (blended).
- One tablespoon of almond oil.
- One tablespoon of finely ground almonds.

Preparation and Use

- Mix blended apricots, almond oil, and ground almonds.
- Apply to your face and neck and leave it on for 10-12 minutes.
- Gently scrub in a circular motion for 3-4 minutes.
- Rinse with warm water.

14. Apple and Cinnamon Clarifying Pack

Ingredients Needed

- One small apple -blended.
- One teaspoon of cinnamon powder.
- Half a teaspoon of powdered sugar.

Preparation and Use

- Mix blended apple with cinnamon and sugar.
- Apply it to your face and leave it on for 10- 12 minutes.
- Gently massage for 2-3 minutes.
- Rinse with cool water.

15. Pear and Honey Hydrating Pack

Ingredients Needed

- Four tablespoons of ripe pear pulp (blended).
- One tablespoon of honey.
- Half a teaspoon of rice flour.

Preparation and Use

- Mix blended pear with honey and rice flour.
- Apply to your face and leave it on for 10-12 minutes.
- Rinse with lukewarm water.

16. Lemon and Egg White Tightening Pack

Ingredients Needed

- One egg white
- One teaspoon of lemon juice

Preparation and Use

- Whip egg white and lemon juice until frothy.
- Apply to your face and leave it on for 7-10 minutes.
- Rinse with cool water.

Before using any of these packs, make sure your face is clean and makeup-free. Apply it on a small area of your skin to check for any adverse reactions. Avoid applying Packs to the sensitive eye area.

After rinsing off the Pack, follow up with your regular skincare routine, including moisturizer and sunscreen.

These homemade fruit-based packs can provide various benefits for your skin, but results may vary based on your skin type and individual preferences.

If you experience any discomfort or irritation, discontinue use and consult a dermatologist.

17. Turmeric and Greek Yogurt Pack

Ingredients Needed

- One teaspoon of turmeric powder
- Two tablespoons of Greek yogurt

Preparation and Use

- Mix turmeric and yogurt, apply to the face, and leave on for 10-12 minutes.
- Rinse with warm water.
- Turmeric has anti-inflammatory properties.

18. Papaya Enzyme Exfoliating Pack

Ingredients Needed

- Four tablespoons of mashed ripe papaya
- One tablespoon of honey

Preparation and Use

- Mix papaya and honey, apply to the face, and leave on for 10-12 minutes.
- Massage gently for 2-3 minutes before rinsing.
- Rinse with cool water.
- Papaya contains enzymes that exfoliate gently.

19. Honey and Yogurt Exfoliating Face Pack

Ingredients Needed

- One tablespoon of honey.
- One tablespoon of plain yogurt.
- One teaspoon of oatmeal powder.

Preparation and Use

- Mix honey, oatmeal powder, and yogurt to a smooth paste.
- Apply to clean face and neck, and leave on for 10-12 minutes.
- Gently massage for 2-3 minutes before rinsing with warm water.
- Honey is moisturizing, and yogurt contains lactic acid for gentle exfoliation.

20. Banana and Avocado Nourishing Face Pack

Ingredients Needed

- Two tablespoons of mashed ripe banana.
- Two tablespoons of mashed ripe avocado.

Preparation and Use

- Mash banana and avocado to make a smooth paste.
- Apply to the face, leave on for 10-12 minutes, and rinse.
- Avocado's healthy fats nourish the skin.

Homemade Moisturizing Face Pack

Ingredients Needed

Three tablespoons of ripe banana (hydrating and nourishing).

One tablespoon of honey (moisturizing and antibacterial).

One tablespoon of plain yogurt (soothing and exfoliating).

Optional: a few drops of olive oil, avocado oil, or almond oil (extra hydration).

Preparation and Use

Gather Supplies: You'll need a clean bowl, a fork for mashing, and a soft brush or your fingers for application.

Mash the Banana: mash the ripe banana until smooth.

Add Honey and yogurt: Add the honey and yogurt to the mashed banana. Mix the ingredients thoroughly until they mix well.

Optional Oil: If you're adding olive oil or avocado oil, do so at this stage and mix well.

Application: Apply this wonderful mixture to your clean face, avoiding the eye area.

Relax: Leave the Pack on for about 15-20 minutes. You can use this time to relax and unwind.

Rinse Off: Gently rinse the Pack off with warm water. Wipe your face dry with a clean towel.

Moisturize: Follow up with your favorite DIY moisturizer to lock in the benefits of the Pack.

Usage: You can use this Pack 1-2 times a week to keep your skin hydrated and nourished.

Chapter 7:
A Fascinating Story of Lipstick

Is lipstick a recent fashion craze? Well, buckle up for a journey through time! It turns out that the love affair with lip color started about **5,000** years ago, with the trailblazing **Sumerians** and **Indus Valley dwellers from India**. From crushed gemstones to **Cleopatra's bug-based** brilliance, join the ride through history as we explore the ancient roots of this beauty staple.

Lipstick is not just makeup; it's a colorful tale that spans civilizations, from the **scented lips of Tang Dynasty China** to the **ochre-painted rituals** of Aboriginal girls in **Australia**. So, get ready to explore the rich, vibrant, and surprising history of lipstick! The Sumerians crushed gemstones and used them to make their faces look fancy, especially around their lips and eyes. Imagine that—gems on your face!

Over in **Egypt, Cleopatra was a trendsetter.** She crushed bugs, turning them into a red color (called carmine) for her lips. In the Indus Valley, ladies used **pieces of ochre** with a special shape to put color on their lips.

Over a thousand years ago, in China, lipsticks were made **from beeswax**, not just to look good but also to protect their lips. Later, during the Tang Dynasty, they **added scented oils** to make their mouths smell nice, too!

In Australia, Aboriginal girls painted their mouths red with ochre as part of their **puberty rituals**. It was a way of marking an important moment in their lives.

Fast forward to 16th-century England. Queen Elizabeth I was all about those bright red lips and a super white face. Back then, they made lipstick from a mix of beeswax and plant stains. But guess what? Only rich ladies and male actors got to wear makeup. The society said no to makeup for respectable women!

Let's peek into a Parisian moment in the 1870s. When an employee of Guerlain, a famous brand, walked down the street and stumbled upon a candlemaker's store. That moment sparked an idea—what if makeup came on a stick? **The first lipstick was born!** It was pink, refillable, and made from deer tallow, castor oil, and beeswax. It is indeed an example of creative thinking!

By the end of the 19th century, Guerlain was making lipstick for everyone. They even made the first commercial lipstick in 1884, covering it in silk paper. It was a mix of deer tallow, castor oil, and beeswax.

In England, people weren't so into makeup for a long time. It was a no-no, especially in the 19th century. They thought it was daring and improper. Reports even warned about the dangers of using lead and vermilion in cosmetics. Yikes!

By 1921, Londoners finally said, "Hey, makeup is totally fine!" It was like a big, fashionable acceptance party.

So, there you have it—the journey of lipstick from ancient times to becoming a must-have for everyone's makeup bag! In the 19th century, the coloring of lipstick relied on Carmine dye extracted from cochineal scale insects indigenous to Mexico and Central America, living on cactus plants. The process involved combining Carmine extract with calcium salts, resulting in usable Carmine dye.

During this era, lipstick application did not involve the familiar tube; instead, it was delicately brushed onto the lips. However, the costliness of Carmine dye and the perceived unnatural and theatrical appearance it imparted led to general disapproval of everyday lipstick use.

They deemed only actors and actresses acceptable to adorn their lips with this colorful cosmetic, and even by 1880, only a few stage actresses dared to wear lipstick in public.

The tide turned as some actresses defied convention by wearing lipstick openly. Before the late 19th century, women restricted the application of makeup to the confines of their homes. By 1912, fashionable American women gradually embraced lipstick, though a New York Times article cautioned on its cautious use. The evolution continued, and by 1915, Maurice Levy introduced cylinder metal containers for selling lipstick.

Women had to skillfully slide a tiny lever on the side of the lipstick tube to access it using the edge of their fingernails. Meanwhile, Europe had already seen push-up metal containers for lipsticks since 1911.

In 1923, a breakthrough came with the patenting of the first swivel-up tube by James Bruce Mason Jr. in Nashville, Tennessee. This innovation marked a pivotal moment as women, now wearing lipstick for photographs, found greater acceptance of this cosmetic. Renowned beauty entrepreneurs Elizabeth Arden and Estee Lauder began retailing lipsticks in their salons, further cementing its popularity among women.

The landscape of lipstick transformed during the Second World War, with metal lipstick tubes making way for plastic and paper alternatives because of shortages in essential ingredients like petroleum and castor oil. Despite the scarcity, the war provided opportunities for women in engineering and scientific research.

In the late 1940s, Hazel Bishop, an organic chemist, revolutionized the industry by creating the first long-lasting lipstick, aptly named No-Smear lipstick. Assisted by Raymond Specter, an advertiser, Bishop's lipstick venture flourished.

Let's now fast forward to the 1990s, and a new era dawned with the invention of a wax-free, semi-permanent liquid formula for lip color by the Lip-Ink International company. This innovative concept inspired other companies to emulate it, leading to the introduction of their versions of long-lasting "lip stain" or "liquid lip color."From its theatrical origins to becoming a staple in every woman's cosmetic kit, the evolution of lipstick stands as a testament to its enduring allure."

Important Tips

Store homemade lip balms in small, clean containers in a cool place to keep them fresh.

You can use the ingredients based on your preferences and the number of lip balm tubes or pots you want to fill.

Ensure that you are not allergic to any of the ingredients used.

Customize the recipes by adjusting the quantities and adding your favorite essential oils for flavor and fragrance. Enjoy the nourishing benefits of these DIY lip balms!

******

Chapter 8: Homemade Lip balms

1. Beeswax and Coconut Oil

Ingredients

- One tablespoon of beeswax pellets.
- One tablespoon of coconut oil.
- Some drops of essential oil (optional for flavor and fragrance).

Preparation

- In a heat-safe container, combine the beeswax pellets and coconut oil.
- Create a double boiler by placing the container in a pot of simmering water.
- Stir the mixture until the beeswax and coconut oil completely melt.
- If you are using essential oil, add some drops to the mixture and stir well.
- Pour it into lip balm tubes or small bottles.
- Let the mixture cool and solidify before using.

2. Shea Butter and Cocoa Butter Lip Balm

Ingredients

- One tablespoon shea butter
- One tablespoon of cocoa butter
- One teaspoon of sweet almond oil

Preparation

- In a heat-safe container, combine the shea butter and cocoa butter.
- Create a double boiler and melt the kinds of butter over low heat.
- Stir in the sweet almond oil.
- After melting and mixing everything, please remove it from the heat.
- Pour the mixture into lip balm tubes or containers.
- Allow the mixture to cool and solidify before using.

3. Honey and Almond Oil Lip Balm

Ingredients

One tablespoon of beeswax pellets

One tablespoon of almond oil

One teaspoon honey

Preparation

In a heat-safe container, combine the beeswax pellets and almond oil.

Create a double boiler and melt the mixture over low heat.

Stir in the honey until well incorporated.

Pour it into lip balm tubes or pots.

Let the mixture cool and solidify before using.

4. Avocado Oil and Peppermint

Ingredients

One tablespoon of avocado oil

One tablespoon of coconut oil

One tablespoon of beeswax pellets

5-10 drops of peppermint essential oil

Preparation

In a heat-safe container, combine the avocado oil, coconut oil, and beeswax pellets.

Create a double boiler and melt the mixture over low heat.

Once melted, add the peppermint essential oil and stir well.

Pour the mixture into tubes or pots.

Allow the mixture to cool and solidify before using.

5. Green Tea and Olive Oil

Ingredients

- One tablespoon of olive oil
- One teaspoon of green tea leaves (finely ground)
- One teaspoon of beeswax pellets

Preparation

- In a heat-safe container, combine the olive oil and green tea leaves.
- Heat the mixture over low heat for about 20 minutes in a double boiler.
- Strain the mixture to remove the green tea leaves.
- Return the infused oil to the heat-safe container and add the beeswax pellets.
- Melt it over low heat, stirring until combined.
- Pour the mixture into tubes or pots.
- Let it cool and solidify before using.

6. Cocoa Powder and Vanilla

Ingredients

- One tablespoon of cocoa butter
- One tablespoon of coconut oil
- One teaspoon of beeswax pellets
- A pinch of cocoa powder
- A few drops of vanilla extract

Preparation

- In a heat-safe container, combine the cocoa butter, coconut oil, and beeswax pellets.
- Create a double boiler and melt the mixture over low heat.
- Stir in a pinch of cocoa powder for color and a few drops of vanilla extract for flavor.
- Pour it into lip balm tubes or pots.
- Let it cool and solidify before using.

7. Rosehip Oil and Lavender

Ingredients

- One tablespoon of rosehip oil
- One tablespoon of beeswax pellets
- 5-10 drops of lavender essential oil

Preparation

- In a heat-safe container, combine the rosehip oil and beeswax pellets.
- Create a double boiler and melt the mixture over low heat.
- Add the lavender oil and stir well.
- Pour it into lip balm tubes or pots.
- Let it cool and solidify before using.

8. Honey and Lemon

Ingredients

- One tablespoon of beeswax pellets
- One tablespoon of sweet almond oil
- One teaspoon honey
- A few drops of lemon essential oil

Preparation

- In a heat-safe container, combine the beeswax pellets and sweet almond oil.
- Create a double boiler and melt the mixture over low heat.
- Stir in the honey and a few drops of lemon essential oil.
- Pour it into lip balm tubes or pots.
- Let it cool and solidify before using.

9. Coconut Oil and Chamomile

Ingredients

- One tablespoon of coconut oil
- One teaspoon of chamomile flowers (dried and finely ground)
- One teaspoon of beeswax pellets

Preparation

- In a heat-safe container, combine the coconut oil and chamomile flowers.
- Heat the mixture over low heat for about 15 - 20 minutes in a double boiler.
- Strain the mixture to remove the chamomile flowers.
- Return the infused oil to the heat-safe container and add the beeswax pellets.
- Melt it over low heat, stirring until combined.
- Pour it into lip balm tubes or pots.
- Let it cool and solidify before using.

10. Mango Butter and Vanilla

Ingredients

- One tablespoon of mango butter
- One tablespoon of coconut oil
- One teaspoon of beeswax pellets
- A few drops of vanilla extract

Preparation

- In a heat-safe container, combine the mango butter, coconut oil, and beeswax pellets.
- Create a double boiler and melt the mixture over low heat.
- Add a few drops of vanilla essence for flavor.
- Pour it into lip balm tubes or pots.

******

Chapter 9:

Timeless Beauty- Easy-to-Make Anti-Aging Creams

Aging is a fact of life. Looking your age is not. -Dr Howard Murad.

Introduction

The process of aging is inevitable, and one of its most noticeable manifestations is the gradual loss of skin elasticity, leading to sagging. As we grow, our skin undergoes a complex interplay of biological processes and external influences that contribute to its changing structure and appearance.

Understanding why our skin becomes saggy with age requires a closer look at the intricate mechanisms involving collagen, elastin, and various environmental factors that shape the aging process.

At the core of youthful skin lies a protein-rich matrix, primarily composed of collagen and elastin fibers, providing the foundation for its firmness and resilience. Collagen, likened to the scaffolding of a building, maintains the skin's structural integrity, ensuring it remains taut and supple.

Elastin is the elastic fiber that allows the skin to stretch and recoil, like a rubber band. Together, these proteins create a dynamic support system that keeps the skin buoyant and capable of adapting to facial expressions and movements.

However, as the years unfold, this intricate matrix undergoes a gradual transformation, and the telltale signs of aging become increasingly apparent. The primary culprit behind sagging skin is the natural depletion of collagen and elastin. The body's collagen production peaks in our early twenties and gradually declines after that.

Environmental factors, lifestyle choices, and genetic predispositions exacerbated this decline. With reduced collagen levels, the skin loses its firmness and succumbs to the effects of gravity. It further leads to saggy and wrinkled skin.

The degradation of elastin further amplifies the sagging phenomenon. Elastin fibers are essential for the skin's ability to retain its shape after stretching or contracting. Over time, these fibers become less resilient and lose their elasticity, compromising the skin's ability to bounce back. The combined impact of reduced collagen and elastin levels results in a loss of structural support, creating an environment conducive to sagging.

Another key contributor to sagging skin is the gradual decrease in **hyaluronic acid production. Hyaluronic**

acid is a natural substance in the skin that maintains skin hydration and plumpness. As its production diminishes, the skin becomes more prone to dryness and loses its ability to retain water, further exacerbating the appearance of sagging.

While intrinsic factors, such as genetics, play a significant role in the aging process, extrinsic factors also wield considerable influence. Sun exposure stands out as a major external factor contributing to sagging skin.

Ultraviolet (UV) rays of the sun p trigger the breakdown of collagen and elastin fibers. This process, known as **photoaging**, accelerates the natural aging of the skin, hastening the onset of sagging and wrinkles. Too much-unprotected exposure to the sun's harmful rays becomes a major factor that significantly contributes to the premature aging of the skin.

Lifestyle choices such as smoking and poor nutrition can speed up the aging process and contribute to sagging skin. Smoking, in particular, is notorious for its detrimental effects on collagen and elastin, impairing the skin's ability to regenerate and repair itself. A diet devoid of essential nutrients and antioxidants can also deprive the skin of the support it needs to maintain its vitality and resilience.

Why do we get wrinkles on the face and neck?

The development of wrinkles on the face and neck is a natural part of the aging process, influenced by a combination of intrinsic and extrinsic factors. Understanding the causes and implementing preventive measures, including natural remedies, can contribute to delaying the onset and reducing the severity of wrinkles.

One of the primary contributors to facial and neck wrinkles is the gradual loss of collagen and elastin, proteins crucial for the skin's structure and elasticity. As we age, the production of these proteins decreases, reducing skin firmness and resilience. **Repeated facial expressions** such as smiling, squinting, and frowning contribute to the formation of dynamic wrinkles—lines that appear during facial expressions and become more pronounced.

Sun exposure, a major extrinsic factor, plays a significant role in the development of wrinkles. Ultraviolet (UV) rays of the sun affect the skin, damaging collagen and elastin fibers. This damage weakens the skin's support structure, accelerating the formation of wrinkles and fine lines. Prolonged exposure to afternoon sun without protection can lead to premature aging, making sun protection a crucial element in wrinkle prevention.

Secrets to Delay Wrinkles

Sun Protection

Using sunglasses, umbrellas, and broad hats can save your face and neck from harsh sun rays. Use sunscreen with a good amount of SPF to protect your skin from harmful UV rays. Apply it generously to the face, neck, and other exposed areas, and reapply every two hours, especially when outdoors.

Avoid Smoking

Smoking speeds up the aging process and contributes to the formation of wrinkles. Giving up smoking can have a major benefit for your skin's health and overall well-being.

Hydration

Keep your skin well-hydrated by drinking an adequate amount of water. Moisturized skin is less prone to wrinkles.

Healthy Diet

Have a balanced diet rich in antioxidants, vitamins, and minerals. These nutrients support skin health and protect against oxidative stress, a contributor to premature aging.

Aloe Vera:

Aloe Vera has soothing properties that hydrate and nourish the skin and reduce the appearance of wrinkles and fine lines.

Gentle Skincare.

Use a gentle homemade cleanser and avoid harsh skincare products that can devour the skin of its natural oils. Moisturize regularly to maintain skin hydration.

Natural Remedies to Delay Skin Wrinkles

Coconut Oil:

This natural moisturizer contains antioxidants and promotes collagen production. Apply a small amount to the face and neck regularly.

Green Tea Extract:

Green tea is rich in antioxidants, which can help protect the skin from oxidative stress. Applying cooled green tea bags to the skin gives excellent results.

Vitamin C:

Adding foods rich in vitamin C into your diet or using skincare products containing this vitamin are helpful. Vitamin C promotes collagen synthesis and helps combat free radicals.

Face Massage:

Gently massaging the face and neck can improve blood circulation and stimulate collagen production. Use upward and outward motions to avoid tugging on the skin.

Yogurt Mask:

Apply a mixture of yogurt and honey to the face as a natural mask. Yogurt contains lactic acid, which can exfoliate the skin, while honey provides moisture.

Omega-3 Fatty Acids:

Include foods rich in omega-3 fatty acids, such as fish, flaxseeds, and walnuts, in your diet. These fatty acids support skin health and hydration.

Conclusion

The phenomenon of sagging skin and wrinkles as we age is a multifaceted interplay of intrinsic and extrinsic factors. The gradual decline in collagen and elastin, coupled with the diminishing production of hyaluronic acid, sets the stage for losing skin firmness and elasticity. Environmental influences, especially sun exposure, further speed up this process, making sagging skin a visible marker of passing time. While the aging process is inevitable, understanding the mechanisms behind sagging skin empowers individuals to make informed choices in their skincare routines and lifestyles, potentially slowing down the visible effects of aging and promoting skin health and vibrancy.

While wrinkles are a natural part of aging, adopting a comprehensive approach to skincare, healthy lifestyle choices, and incorporating natural remedies can contribute to maintaining youthful and resilient skin. Consistency in these practices is key to achieving long-term benefits and promoting overall skin health.

Homemade Nourishing Night Cream for Face and Neck

Ingredients Required

- Two tablespoons of shea butter or cocoa butter.
- One tablespoon of coconut oil.
- One teaspoon of jojoba oil or almond oil.
- One teaspoon of rosehip seed oil or rose essential oil.
- 5-7 drops of lavender essential oil (optional for fragrance.

Benefits of Each Ingredient

Shea Butter / Cocoa butter: Deeply moisturizes, soothes, and promotes skin elasticity. Rich in vitamins and fatty acids.

Coconut Oil: Provides hydration, has anti-inflammatory properties, and contains antioxidants for overall skin health.

Jojoba Oil: Balances oil production, deeply moisturizes without clogging pores, and contains vitamin E and B-complex vitamins.

Rosehip Seed Oil: Packed with antioxidants and essential fatty acids, it helps reduce fine lines and scars and promotes skin regeneration.

Lavender Essential Oil: Optional for a calming fragrance. Lavender oil also has soothing and anti-inflammatory properties.

Preparation and Use

- Melt Shea Butter in a heat-safe bowl, using a double boiler, until it turns into liquid.
- Then add the coconut oil to the melted shea butter and mix well until combined.
- Mix in the jojoba oil and rosehip seed oil, ensuring a smooth and consistent texture.
- If you desire a pleasant scent and additional soothing properties, add 5-7 drops of lavender essential oil. Mix well.
- Let it cool to room temperature and set.
- You may speed up the process by placing it in the refrigerator for a short time.

Whipping (Optional):

For a lighter texture, you can whip the partially set mixture using a hand mixer or a whisk until it becomes fluffy.

Storage:

Transfer the night cream to a clean, airtight jar. Store it in a cool, dark place to preserve the integrity of the natural ingredients.

Usage:

Apply a small amount of the night cream to your face and neck after your evening skincare routine. Massage gently in upward motions.

Shelf Life:

Use this cream within 2-3 months. Keep an eye out for any changes in scent or consistency, and discard if you notice any signs of spoilage.

Benefits of the Nourishing Night Cream

Deep Hydration:

Shea butter and coconut oil provide intense hydration, combating dryness.

Anti-aging Properties:

Jojoba and rosehip seed oils contribute to reducing signs of aging and promoting skin regeneration.

Balanced Moisture:

Jojoba oil helps balance the skin's natural oil production, making it suitable for various skin types.

Please Note:

Perform a patch test before applying the night cream to ensure you don't have any adverse reactions. Adjust the essential oil quantity based on personal preference and skin sensitivity. If you have allergies or skin conditions, please consult with a dermatologist before trying any homemade cosmetics.

Benefits of Facial Massage

Rejuvenate Your Skin and Spirit with Facial Massage

In our fast-paced modern world, stress is inevitable and has become a part of daily life, affecting our mental and physical well-being. As a result, self-care practices that promote relaxation and rejuvenation have become essential components of maintaining a balanced and healthy lifestyle.

Among these practices, facial massage has emerged as a popular and effective way to enhance the skin's appearance and provide a soothing escape from the pressures of daily life. With its roots deeply embedded in ancient wellness traditions, facial massage offers a holistic approach to skincare that addresses beauty's outer and inner aspects.

Benefits of Facial Massage: Nurturing the Skin and Beyond

Facial massage is not merely a luxury indulgence; it offers many advantages that span from the physical to the emotional. This practice, often characterized by gentle and deliberate touch, can transform your skin and elevate your overall well-being. Let's explore some benefits of incorporating facial massage into your self-care routine:

Improved Blood Circulation and Lymphatic Drainage

The rhythmic motions of facial massage stimulate blood flow, allowing oxygen and essential nutrients to reach the skin's surface. Improved circulation contributes to a healthy, radiant complexion.

Active 2: The enhancement of lymphatic drainage helps in removing toxins and reducing facial puffiness. This process helps sculpt the face, resulting in a more defined and youthful appearance.

Relaxation and Stress Relief

One of the most notable benefits of facial massage is its relaxation and ease of stress. The gentle touch and soothing movements calm the nervous system, allowing you to unwind and escape from the pressures of the day. Massage helps release tension in facial muscles and leads to an overall sense of relaxation, affecting your mental, physical, and emotional well-being.

Muscle Tone and Facial Contouring

Regular facial massages can promote muscle tone and elasticity, preventing or at least delaying the formation of wrinkles.

By targeting specific facial muscles, such as those along the jawline and cheekbones, facial massage improves facial contouring and a more sculpted appearance.

Enhanced Product Absorption

Performing a facial massage using skincare products can significantly enhance their absorption into the skin.

The gentle kneading and tapping motions help the products penetrate deeper, maximizing their effectiveness and providing optimal hydration.

Natural Face-Lifting Effect

The skin's elasticity diminishes as we age, leading to sagging and loss of firmness. Facial massage can help counteract these effects by stimulating collagen production and promoting skin tightening.

The increased blood flow and muscle engagement contribute to a natural face-lifting effect, leaving you with a revitalized and more youthful appearance.

Mind-Body Connection

Facial massage isn't just about pampering the skin; it also fosters a deeper connection between the mind and body.

The meditative quality of the massage encourages mindfulness, allowing you to be fully present in the moment and promoting a sense of inner peace.

Release of Jaw Tension

Many people carry tension in their jaw due to stress or teeth grinding. Facial massage can help alleviate this tension and promote relaxation in the jaw muscles.

By releasing jaw tension, you can experience relief from headaches and discomfort and even improve your sleep quality.

Boosted Self-Confidence

Taking the time to care for your skin and engage in self-care practices can positively impact your self-confidence and self-esteem.

The glow and radiance following a facial massage can boost your sense of self-worth, helping you feel more comfortable and confident in your skin.

In conclusion, facial massage is a multifaceted practice that transcends the boundaries of skincare alone. Its benefits extend beyond aesthetics, physical health, emotional well-being, and self-care. By embracing this ancient ritual, you embark on a journey to rejuvenate your skin and spirit. As you gently caress your face, you nurture your inner self, creating a harmonious balance that radiates outward and inward. So, treat yourself to the gift of facial massage and discover a path to enhanced vitality, relaxation, and self-love.

Time to Get Ready

1. Thoroughly wash your hands before starting the massage, and be mindful if you have grown nails.
2. Tie back your hair to keep it away from your face.
3. Create a calm and comfortable environment with soft lighting and soothing music.
4. Apply a homemade, chemical-free, gentle facial oil, moisturizer, or massage cream to provide lubrication for the massage.

DIY Anti-aging Cream for Massage

Ingredients Required

- Almonds -15-20.
- Walnuts -six.
- Almond oil, two teaspoons.
- Vitamin E oil one teaspoon or 6-9 Vitamin E capsules.
- Aloe vera gel, four teaspoons.
- Saffron strands 15-20.
- Rose essential oil four drops (optional).
- Rosewater -three to four tablespoons.

Shelf life: It lasts about two weeks if stored in a refrigerator

Preparation and Use

- Soak almonds and walnuts separately in water for 4-5 hours (later discard this water.
- Soak saffron strands in 2-3 spoons of rosewater.
- Peel almonds and grind them with walnuts to a fine, smooth paste by adding rosewater.
- Add rosewater little by little, or else the mixture will become watery. Strain the mixture using a fine-meshed strainer or a thin cotton cloth. (We can use the residue as a scrub.

- Add almond oil. Vitamin E oil and soaked saffron to the strained liquid. Mix well.
- Add Aloe vera gel and rose essential oil to the mixture and mix it thoroughly to avoid lumps.
- Store it in a clean container and store it in the refrigerator.
- Apply it on your face daily, and you can also use this cream for facial massages.
- This fragrant cream makes your skin soft and radiant.

Step-by-Step Techniques for Facial Massage

If you follow the instructions given here, you will have a great facial massage at home without depending on others and spending no money.

Massage Your Forehead

1. Begin the facial massage in the middle of your forehead area using your fingertips to make small circular movements.
2. Gradually move outwards towards the temples.
3. Repeat it several times to relieve tension.

Massage Your Temples

1. Use your thumbs to press gently and rotate in small circles on the temples to relieve stress.
2. Apply mild, controlled pressure and release that pressure gently and rhythmically.
3. Spend a few moments at each temple to promote relaxation.

Massaging Eye Area

1. The ring finger is the weakest. Using the ring fingers ensures gentle pressure.
2. Lightly massage around the eye sockets with your ring fingers, starting at the inner corners and moving outward.
3. Be very gentle when you massage around the delicate skin of the eyes.
4. Repeat this motion a few times to reduce puffiness.

Massage Your Cheeks

1. Make upward sweeping motions from the jawline towards the cheekbones with your fingers and palms.
2. Use gentle pressure and repeat these movements several times.
3. It helps improve blood circulation and tone the facial muscles.

Massage Your Nose

1. Using your index fingers, trace the bridge of your nose from top to bottom.
2. Apply slight pressure and move in a straight line.
3. It relieves tension in the nasal area and helps sinus drainage.

Massage Your Jawline

1. Place your thumbs under your chin and use your fingers to support the sides of your face. Apply gentle upward strokes along the jawline, moving towards the ears.
2. Repeat this motion to help relax the jaw muscles.

Massage Your Mouth Area

1. Use your index and middle fingers on both sides of your mouth area to massage the area around your lips in circular motions.
2. Be gentle, as the skin around the mouth is sensitive.

Massage Your Neck and Collarbone

1. Extend the massage to your neck and collarbone (clavicle) area.
2. Use upward strokes with your fingers to ease tension.
3. Avoid applying excessive pressure on the neck and massage gently.

Finish

1. Take a few deep breaths to help you relax further.
2. Use your palms to press the entire face gently, holding for a few seconds.
3. It can help the moisturizer used during the massage to be absorbed better.

Post-Massage:

1. With a clean cotton pad, gently wipe off any excess oil or cream from your face.
2. Hydrate yourself by drinking water to maintain skin hydration.
3. Avoid exposing your skin to harsh sunlight immediately after the massage.

Everyone's skin is different, so adjusting the pressure and techniques is essential based on your comfort level. If you have any skin conditions or concerns, it's a good idea to consult a dermatologist before performing a facial massage.

Chapter 10: Holistic Approach to Glowing Skin

Achieving radiant skin goes beyond external applications and treatments. It is all about adapting and practicing holistic well-being.

A holistic approach to radiant skin encompasses various aspects of our lifestyle, including skincare practices, stress-free living, mindful exercises, balanced nutrition, and adequate hydration. Drink plenty of water to keep your skin healthy. Water flushes out toxins from the body and helps maintain skin hydration.

Applying cosmetics alone without taking a holistic approach is like painting cracked furniture. We must take a holistic approach. Any form of exercise or dancing, cycling, aerobics or swimming is essential to maintain good health.

Let's understand the components of a holistic skincare routine that can contribute to achieving that coveted radiant glow.

Yoga Mudras for Skin Health:

Yoga, propounded by Maharshi Patanjali, is India's offering to the global community. Yoga is not just about stretching and bending exercises; it goes much beyond physical fitness.

It promotes physical fitness, encourages mental peace, and aids in the quest for the ultimate truth of human existence. It is a way of caring for your mind, body, and spirit. And now, it's gained popularity worldwide because it is beneficial to all with no strings attached to it.

Besides those Yoga poses that work your whole body, there's something else you should know -about yoga mudras. These are like unique hand gestures that can do amazing things for your health.

I'm introducing you to two Yoga Mudras that are beneficial to reduce stress and keep our skin healthy. I will soon publish a book on Yoga Mudras and Pranayama, which will be a comprehensive guide for complete healthcare.

1. Gyan Mudra (Knowledge Seal):

The Gyan Mudra involves touching the tip of the index finger to the tip of the thumb, creating a circular shape. This mudra is believed to improve concentration and mental clarity, reducing stress that can contribute to skin issues. A calm mind often reflects in a radiant complexion.

Gyan Mudra is also called Chin Mudra. Gyan is a Sanskrit word for **knowledge,** and this Mudra is excellent for strengthening memory.

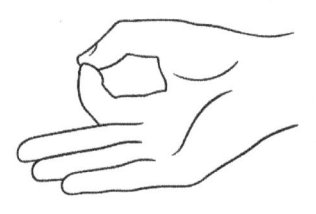

Method

- Keep the palms facing upwards on your knee and sit erect.
- Bend the index finger and touch the tip of your thumb gently.
- Focus on the area of contact of the fingers.
- You can perform this from twenty minutes to thirty minutes.

Benefits

1. It relieves anxiety and stress and calms your mind.
2. It boosts overall well-being.
3. It promotes healthy skin.
4. It also controls hair fall and helps hair growth.
5. It balances body hormones.
6. It gives excellent results when practiced after breakfast and lunch.

2. Prithvi Mudra (Earth Seal):

It is formed by touching the ring finger to the tip of the thumb. Prithvi Mudra is associated with the Earth element. This mudra enhances the body's connection to the Earth's energy, promoting skin health and vitality.

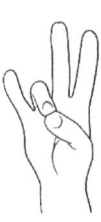

Prithvi means the earth in Sanskrit. Prithvi Mudra balances the earth element in our body. This Mudra promotes glowing skin.

Method

1. Bend the ring finger towards your thumb and touch the tip of your thumb with that of your ring finger.
2. Hold it gently and stay in this position for at least thirty minutes, and you may extend the time to forty-five minutes. Keep other fingers straight. Practice it twice a day for better results.

Benefits

- This gesture is good for your skin's health. It calms down your mind. It also controls dandruff and promotes a healthy scalp.

Breathing Exercises (Pranayama) for Skin:

In Sanskrit, *Prana* refers to life or "cosmic energy" or breath, and *Ayama* means "to control." So, the literal meaning of *Pranayama* (*Pranasya Ayamaha*) is "controlled breathing".

Pranayama is a part of Yoga Practices. Breathing is a necessity for all living creatures. *Pranayama* cleans the body, mind, and spirit, promoting good health.

Pranayama is a term from yoga that refers to the practice of breath control. It involves various techniques to manipulate the breath to enhance physical and mental well-being.

Pranayama techniques include conscious regulation of inhalation, exhalation, and retention of breath. Practitioners believe that by controlling the breath, they can influence the flow of prana in the body, promoting balance and harmony. It is an integral part of many yoga traditions and is a preparation for meditation.

Anuloma Viloma (Alternate Nostril Breathing):

Anuloma Viloma involves breathing through one nostril at a time, promoting balance in the body's energy flow. This Pranayama reduces stress and enhances circulation, contributing to healthier skin.

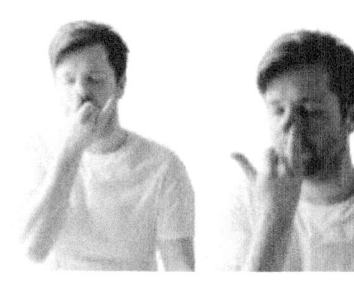

- Exhale completely.
- Close the right nostril and inhale through the left nostril.
- Then, close the left nostril and open the right nostril.
- Breathe out slowly through the right nostril, then slowly breathe in through the right nostril.
- Close the right nostril, and breathe out through the left nostril.
- It completes one cycle. Begin with five repetitions or cycles and gradually increase to 20 cycles per session over ten days.

Homemade Moisturizers, Toners, and Face Packs:

1. **Moisturizer:** Create a simple moisturizer by combining equal parts of coconut oil and aloe vera gel. Coconut oil nourishes the skin, while aloe vera provides hydration without clogging pores. This natural blend can be applied to the face and body for a moisture boost.

2. **Toner:** Green tea makes an excellent toner because of its antioxidant properties. Brew green tea, let it cool, and use it as a toner to tighten pores and reduce inflammation. It's a refreshing addition to your skincare routine.

3. **Face Pack:** Mix honey, yogurt, and a pinch of turmeric to create a hydrating and anti-inflammatory face pack. Honey moisturizes, yogurt exfoliates gently, and turmeric reduces inflammation, leaving your skin radiant and refreshed.

This book features many recipes for natural skincare cosmetics. You may choose the one you like and try them all by rotating them.

Balanced Diet and Hydration:

A well-balanced diet rich in vitamins, minerals, and antioxidants is crucial for radiant skin. Include a variety of fruits, vegetables, whole grains, and lean proteins in your meals. Foods like berries, leafy greens, and fatty fish contribute to skin health.

Hydration is equally important. Drinking an adequate amount of water helps flush out toxins and keeps the skin hydrated from within. Herbal teas and infused water with slices of cucumber or lemon are excellent choices.

Sun Protection:

Protecting your skin from the sun is a non-negotiable part of any holistic skincare routine. Use a sunscreen with at least SPF 30, even on cloudy days. Wearing hats and sunglasses can provide extra protection against harmful UV rays.

Mindful Practices:

Stress and lack of sleep can negatively affect the skin. Incorporate mindfulness practices such as meditation and deep breathing into your routine to manage stress levels. Quality sleep is essential for skin repair and regeneration, so aim for 7-9 hours of restful sleep each night.

Exercise for Radiant Skin:

Regular physical activity promotes blood circulation, delivering essential nutrients to the skin and flushing out toxins. Choose exercises you enjoy, whether it's yoga, jogging, or dancing, to keep your body and skin healthy.

Conclusion:

A holistic approach to radiant skin involves a harmonious blend of skincare practices, mindful exercises, a balanced diet, and proper hydration. Incorporating yoga mudras and Pranayama enhances the mind-body connection, contributing to overall well-being. Homemade moisturizers, toners, and face packs provide natural nourishment to the skin, while a balanced diet, hydration, and sun protection are fundamental for maintaining skin health. By adopting these holistic practices, you not only achieve radiant skin but also nurture your overall health and vitality.

******

References

1. A Textbook of Ayurveda (Ayurveda Shiksha) by A Lakshmi Pathi
2. Mudras Yoga with the hands b- Guru Vishnu
3. A Complete Handbook of Nature Cure by H K Bakhru
4. Wikipedia
5. https://www.ncbi.nlm.nih.gov/pmc/articles
6. https://www.researchgate.net/publication/358768633_Lipsticks_History_Formulations_and_Production_A_Narrative_Review
7. https://dermskinco.com/collections/frontpage/products/skin-scripts-hyluronic-acid
8. http://www.current-pharmaceutical-design.com/articles/86775/cytoprotective-polyphenols-against-chronological-skin-aging-and-cutaneous-photodamage

9. https://www.drjamesglutathioneinjection.com/Blog/Dr-James-Glutathione-Injections-for-Skin-Tightening-and-Firming.aspx
10. https://pureformpethealth.com/blogs/pureform-pet-care/fat-soluble-vitamins
11. https://www.celebricious.com/2022/07/introducing-noor-1-your-first-defence-in-fighting-the-signs-of-aging/
12. https://www.newsheads.in/lifestyle/fashion/tips-how-to-protect-lips-during-summer-in-simple-ways-article-14380
13. https://www.chiropracticomaha.com/is-it-possible-to-slow-or-reverse-aging/
14. https://skyntherapyblog.com/about-acne/what-to-do-if-acne-returns-after-accutane/

Made in the USA
Coppell, TX
14 December 2024